DR. BARBARA CURE FOR HIV/AIDS

Unlocking Vibrant Health; Discover Dr.Barbara Transformative Approach To Combat HIV/AIDS Naturally. Explore Proven Methods For Holistic Healing And Renewed Wellness

Felipe Carmen

COPYRIGHT © 2023

All rights reserved. No part of this publication may be reproduced, distributed, or transmitted in any form or by any means, including photocopying, recording, or other electronic or mechanical methods, without the prior written permission of the publisher, except in the case of brief quotations embodied in critical reviews and certain other noncommercial uses permitted by copyright law.

CHAPTER ONE

Introduction to Dr. Barbara's Healing Method: Understanding the Principles of Natural Healing and Immune Support

Dr. Barbara's Healing Method represents a holistic approach to health and well-being, emphasizing natural healing and immune support. Rooted in principles derived from traditional medicine, modern science, and alternative therapies, this method offers a comprehensive framework for individuals seeking to optimize their health and boost their immune system.

At its core, Dr. Barbara's Healing Method recognizes the interconnectedness of the mind, body, and spirit in promoting overall wellness. It acknowledges the body's innate ability to heal itself when provided with the right conditions and support. By understanding and applying the principles of natural healing and immune support, individuals can empower themselves to take charge of their health and achieve greater vitality.

Principles of Natural Healing

Natural healing is based on the belief that the body has an inherent ability to heal itself given the right conditions. This approach emphasizes the use of natural remedies and therapies to support the body's own healing mechanisms. Dr. Barbara's

Healing Method draws upon several key principles of natural healing:

1. **Whole-Person Approach**: Rather than focusing solely on alleviating symptoms, natural healing considers the individual as a whole – encompassing physical, mental, emotional, and spiritual aspects. This holistic perspective recognizes the interconnectedness of various bodily systems and aims to address underlying imbalances.

2. **Nutrition and Diet**: A foundational aspect of natural healing involves nourishing the body with nutrient-dense foods that support optimal health. Emphasizing a diet rich in fruits, vegetables, whole grains, lean proteins, and healthy fats can provide essential vitamins, minerals, and antioxidants necessary for immune function and overall well-being.

3. **Stress Management**: Chronic stress can weaken the immune system and contribute to a host of health problems. Natural healing encourages the adoption of stress-reduction techniques such as mindfulness meditation, deep breathing exercises, yoga, and tai chi to promote relaxation and resilience.

4. **Physical Activity**: Regular exercise is vital for supporting immune function, reducing inflammation, and maintaining overall health. Incorporating a variety of physical activities – including aerobic exercise, strength training, and flexibility

exercises – can enhance immune function and contribute to a sense of well-being.

5. **Sleep Hygiene**: Quality sleep is essential for immune function and overall health. Natural healing emphasizes the importance of establishing healthy sleep habits, such as maintaining a consistent sleep schedule, creating a relaxing bedtime routine, and optimizing sleep environment for restorative rest.

Immune Support Strategies

In addition to principles of natural healing, Dr. Barbara's Healing Method incorporates specific strategies to support and strengthen the immune system. These strategies are designed to enhance the body's natural defenses against pathogens and promote overall immune resilience:

1. **Nutritional Support**: Certain nutrients play key roles in supporting immune function. Dr. Barbara's Healing Method recommends a balanced diet rich in immune-boosting nutrients such as vitamin C, vitamin D, zinc, selenium, and probiotics. These nutrients can be obtained from a variety of foods or supplements, as needed.

2. **Herbal Remedies**: Herbal medicine has been used for centuries to support immune health and enhance the body's ability to fight infections. Dr. Barbara's Healing Method incorporates evidence-based herbal remedies such as

echinacea, elderberry, astragalus, and medicinal mushrooms to bolster immune function and promote overall well-being.

3. **Lifestyle Modifications**: Certain lifestyle factors can either support or compromise immune function. Dr. Barbara's Healing Method encourages individuals to make healthy lifestyle choices such as avoiding tobacco and excessive alcohol consumption, maintaining a healthy weight, and practicing good hygiene habits to reduce the risk of infections.

4. **Stress Reduction**: Chronic stress can suppress immune function and increase susceptibility to illness. Dr. Barbara's Healing Method emphasizes the importance of stress management techniques such as meditation, yoga, massage therapy, and relaxation exercises to reduce stress levels and support immune health.

5. **Environmental Factors**: Environmental toxins and pollutants can have a detrimental effect on immune function. Dr. Barbara's Healing Method advocates for minimizing exposure to environmental toxins by using natural cleaning products, filtering drinking water, reducing air pollution exposure, and supporting environmental conservation efforts.

Conclusion

Dr. Barbara's Healing Method offers a comprehensive approach to natural healing and immune support, integrating principles from traditional medicine, modern science, and alternative therapies. By adopting a holistic perspective and incorporating strategies to nourish the body, manage stress, and strengthen the immune system, individuals can optimize their health and well-being. Through education, empowerment, and personalized support, Dr. Barbara's Healing Method aims to help individuals cultivate vibrant health and resilience in the face of life's challenges.

CHAPTER TWO

Understanding HIV/AIDS: Insights into the Virus, Transmission, and Impact on the Body's Immune System

HIV/AIDS remains one of the most significant public health challenges globally, with millions of people affected by the virus and its associated complications. Understanding HIV/AIDS requires insight into the virus itself, its modes of transmission, and its profound impact on the body's immune system.

The Human Immunodeficiency Virus (HIV)

HIV is a lentivirus, a type of retrovirus that infects cells of the immune system, particularly CD4 T cells, which play a crucial role in coordinating the body's immune response. The virus primarily targets cells with CD4 surface receptors, such as helper T cells, macrophages, and dendritic cells. Once inside the host cell, HIV integrates its genetic material into the cell's DNA, hijacking the cellular machinery to replicate and produce new virus particles.

HIV is classified into two main types: HIV-1 and HIV-2. HIV-1 is the predominant strain worldwide and is responsible for the majority of HIV infections globally. HIV-2 is less prevalent and is primarily found in West Africa, although cases have been reported in other regions as well.

Transmission of HIV

HIV is transmitted through specific bodily fluids that contain high concentrations of the virus, including blood, semen, vaginal fluids, rectal fluids, and breast milk. The most common modes of HIV transmission include:

1. **Unprotected Sexual Contact**: HIV can be transmitted through unprotected vaginal, anal, or oral sex with an infected partner, particularly if there are open sores, cuts, or mucous membrane tears present.

2. **Sharing of Needles or Syringes**: Injection drug use carries a high risk of HIV transmission if needles or syringes are shared among individuals who are infected.

3. **Mother-to-Child Transmission**: HIV can be passed from an infected mother to her baby during pregnancy, childbirth, or breastfeeding. However, the risk of transmission can be significantly reduced with antiretroviral therapy (ART) during pregnancy and breastfeeding.

4. **Blood Transfusion or Organ Transplant**: While rare in regions with stringent blood screening protocols, HIV can be transmitted through contaminated blood transfusions or organ transplants.

5. **Occupational Exposure**: Healthcare workers may be at risk of HIV transmission through accidental needle sticks or exposure to infected blood or bodily fluids.

Impact on the Immune System

HIV targets and gradually depletes CD4 T cells, which are essential for orchestrating the body's immune response against pathogens. As the virus replicates and spreads throughout the body, it progressively undermines the immune system's ability to mount an effective defense, leading to immunodeficiency.

The immune system's decline in HIV-infected individuals is characterized by several stages:

1. **Acute HIV Infection**: Following initial exposure to the virus, individuals may experience flu-like symptoms, such as fever, fatigue, sore throat, swollen lymph nodes, and rash, during the acute phase of infection. HIV replicates rapidly during this stage, but the immune system typically mounts an initial response.

2. **Chronic HIV Infection**: Without treatment, HIV infection progresses to the chronic stage, characterized by persistent viral replication and gradual depletion of CD4 T cells. As CD4 T cell counts decline, individuals become increasingly susceptible to opportunistic infections and other complications.

3. **AIDS (Acquired Immunodeficiency Syndrome)**: AIDS is the most advanced stage of HIV infection, marked by severe immunodeficiency and the occurrence of opportunistic infections or HIV-related malignancies. The definition of AIDS includes a CD4 T cell count below 200 cells/mm³ or the presence of specific AIDS-defining illnesses.

Conclusion

HIV/AIDS remains a significant global health challenge, with profound implications for affected individuals and communities. Understanding the virus, its modes of transmission, and its impact on the immune system is crucial for developing effective prevention strategies, expanding access to testing and treatment, and combating stigma and discrimination associated with the disease. With continued efforts in research, education, and public health initiatives, progress can be made towards reducing the burden of HIV/AIDS and improving outcomes for those affected by the virus.

CHAPTER THREE

The Role of Nutrition in HIV/AIDS Management: Exploring Dr. Barbara's Herbal Approach to Immune Support

Nutrition plays a vital role in the management of HIV/AIDS, as it directly impacts the immune system, overall health, and quality of life of individuals living with the virus. Dr. Barbara's Herbal Approach to Immune Support offers a holistic perspective on nutrition, emphasizing the importance of a balanced diet and incorporating specific herbs and supplements to bolster immune function and support optimal health in HIV/AIDS management.

Nutritional Considerations in HIV/AIDS

Individuals living with HIV/AIDS often face unique nutritional challenges that can compromise their immune function and overall well-being. These challenges may include:

1. **Increased Nutrient Requirements**: HIV infection can increase the body's nutrient requirements due to factors such as chronic inflammation, metabolic changes, and increased energy expenditure. Adequate intake of essential nutrients is crucial for supporting immune function, maintaining lean body mass, and preventing nutrient deficiencies.

2. **Gastrointestinal Symptoms**: HIV/AIDS and certain medications used in its treatment can cause gastrointestinal

symptoms such as nausea, diarrhea, and loss of appetite, which may interfere with nutrient absorption and lead to malnutrition.

3. **Weight Loss and Wasting**: HIV-associated weight loss and wasting syndrome, known as HIV-associated wasting, can result in the loss of muscle mass and fat tissue, leading to nutritional deficiencies and compromised immune function.

4. **Opportunistic Infections**: Opportunistic infections, common in individuals with advanced HIV/AIDS, can further increase nutrient requirements and contribute to malnutrition.

Dr. Barbara's Herbal Approach to Immune Support

Dr. Barbara's Herbal Approach to Immune Support integrates principles of traditional herbal medicine with modern nutritional science to provide comprehensive support for individuals living with HIV/AIDS. This approach emphasizes the following key elements:

1. **Immune-Boosting Herbs**: Certain herbs have been traditionally used to support immune function and enhance the body's ability to fight infections. Dr. Barbara's approach may incorporate immune-boosting herbs such as echinacea, astragalus, elderberry, and medicinal mushrooms like reishi and shiitake. These herbs contain bioactive compounds that

have been shown to modulate immune responses and support overall health.

2. **Nutrient-Rich Foods**: A balanced diet rich in nutrient-dense foods is essential for individuals living with HIV/AIDS. Dr. Barbara's approach emphasizes the consumption of whole foods such as fruits, vegetables, lean proteins, whole grains, and healthy fats to provide essential vitamins, minerals, antioxidants, and phytonutrients necessary for immune function and overall health.

3. **Supplementation**: In addition to dietary sources, targeted supplementation may be recommended to address specific nutrient deficiencies or support immune function. Dr. Barbara's approach may include supplements such as vitamin C, vitamin D, zinc, selenium, and omega-3 fatty acids, which have been shown to have immune-boosting properties and may benefit individuals living with HIV/AIDS.

4. **Individualized Care**: Dr. Barbara's Herbal Approach to Immune Support recognizes that each individual living with HIV/AIDS may have unique nutritional needs and health concerns. Therefore, care is personalized to address specific nutritional deficiencies, symptoms, and treatment goals.

Conclusion

Nutrition plays a crucial role in the management of HIV/AIDS, impacting immune function, overall health, and quality of life. Dr.

Barbara's Herbal Approach to Immune Support offers a holistic perspective on nutrition, emphasizing the importance of a balanced diet, immune-boosting herbs, targeted supplementation, and personalized care for individuals living with HIV/AIDS. By addressing nutritional needs and supporting immune function, this approach aims to optimize health outcomes and enhance quality of life for those affected by the virus.

CHAPTER FOUR

Herbal Remedies for HIV/AIDS: Identifying Key Herbs and Supplements Recommended by Dr. Barbara

Dr. Barbara's approach to managing HIV/AIDS integrates traditional herbal remedies with modern medical knowledge to provide comprehensive support for individuals living with the virus. Herbal remedies offer a natural and holistic approach to immune support, symptom management, and overall well-being in HIV/AIDS care. Dr. Barbara recommends specific herbs and supplements based on their immune-boosting properties, antiviral effects, and potential to enhance quality of life for individuals affected by HIV/AIDS.

Key Herbs Recommended by Dr. Barbara

1. **Echinacea**: Echinacea is a popular herb known for its immune-stimulating properties. It has been traditionally used to support the body's defense mechanisms and enhance immune function. Echinacea may help strengthen the immune system's response to infections and reduce the severity and duration of colds and other respiratory infections. In HIV/AIDS management, echinacea may be used to support overall immune health and resilience.

2. **Astragalus**: Astragalus is a traditional Chinese herb valued for its immune-modulating and adaptogenic properties. It contains polysaccharides and other bioactive compounds that have been shown to enhance immune function, increase white blood cell counts, and support the body's ability to fight infections. Astragalus may help boost immunity and improve overall vitality in individuals living with HIV/AIDS.

3. **Elderberry**: Elderberry is rich in antioxidants and flavonoids that possess antiviral and immune-enhancing properties. It has been traditionally used to treat colds, flu, and respiratory infections. Elderberry may help reduce the severity and duration of viral infections by inhibiting viral replication and stimulating immune responses. In HIV/AIDS management, elderberry may support immune function and alleviate symptoms associated with viral infections.

4. **Medicinal Mushrooms**: Certain medicinal mushrooms, such as reishi (Ganoderma lucidum), shiitake (Lentinula edodes), and maitake (Grifolafrondosa), have been valued for their immune-modulating and antiviral effects. These mushrooms contain beta-glucans, polysaccharides, and other bioactive compounds that can enhance immune function, increase white blood cell activity, and improve overall immune responses. In HIV/AIDS management, medicinal mushrooms

may help support immune health and reduce the risk of infections.

Supplements Recommended by Dr. Barbara

1. **Vitamin C**: Vitamin C is a powerful antioxidant that plays a crucial role in supporting immune function and reducing oxidative stress. It is involved in the production of white blood cells and antibodies, which are essential for fighting infections. Vitamin C supplementation may help enhance immune responses and reduce the risk of infections in individuals living with HIV/AIDS.

2. **Vitamin D**: Vitamin D is important for immune regulation and may help modulate immune responses in individuals with HIV/AIDS. Adequate vitamin D levels have been associated with reduced risk of respiratory infections and improved immune function. Vitamin D supplementation may be beneficial for individuals with HIV/AIDS, especially those at risk of vitamin D deficiency due to limited sun exposure or impaired absorption.

3. **Zinc**: Zinc is an essential mineral that plays a key role in immune function, wound healing, and protein synthesis. Zinc deficiency is common in individuals with HIV/AIDS and may contribute to immune dysfunction and increased susceptibility to infections. Zinc supplementation may help support immune health, reduce the severity and duration of

infections, and improve overall nutritional status in individuals living with HIV/AIDS.

4. **Selenium**: Selenium is a trace mineral with antioxidant properties that is essential for immune function and cellular health. Selenium deficiency has been associated with immune dysfunction and increased risk of opportunistic infections in individuals with HIV/AIDS. Selenium supplementation may help boost immune responses, reduce oxidative stress, and support overall health in individuals living with the virus.

Conclusion

Herbal remedies and supplements recommended by Dr. Barbara offer natural and holistic support for individuals living with HIV/AIDS. These herbs and supplements are selected based on their immune-boosting properties, antiviral effects, and potential to enhance overall health and well-being in HIV/AIDS management. When used as part of a comprehensive care plan, herbal remedies and supplements can help support immune function, alleviate symptoms, and improve quality of life for individuals affected by the virus. However, it is essential to consult with a healthcare professional before starting any herbal remedies or supplements, especially for individuals with underlying health conditions or those taking medications.

CHAPTER FIVE

Lifestyle Modifications for Immune Support: Strategies for Stress Reduction, Sleep, and Exercise

Lifestyle modifications play a crucial role in supporting immune function and overall well-being. Dr. Barbara emphasizes the importance of incorporating healthy lifestyle habits to enhance immune support, reduce inflammation, and promote resilience against infections. Key strategies for stress reduction, sleep improvement, and regular exercise are integral components of Dr. Barbara's approach to immune support.

Stress Reduction Strategies

Chronic stress can have detrimental effects on immune function, increasing susceptibility to infections and inflammatory conditions. Dr. Barbara recommends the following stress reduction strategies to promote immune support:

1. **Mindfulness Meditation**: Mindfulness meditation involves focusing attention on the present moment without judgment, which can help reduce stress, anxiety, and negative emotions. Regular meditation practice has been shown to improve immune function and enhance resilience to stress.

2. **Deep Breathing Exercises**: Deep breathing exercises, such as diaphragmatic breathing or belly breathing, can activate the body's relaxation response, leading to decreased heart rate, blood pressure, and muscle tension. Deep breathing techniques are effective tools for managing stress and promoting relaxation.

3. **Yoga and Tai Chi**: Yoga and tai chi are mind-body practices that combine gentle movements, controlled breathing, and meditation to promote physical and mental well-being. These practices can help reduce stress, improve flexibility, balance, and coordination, and enhance immune function.

4. **Nature Walks and Outdoor Activities**: Spending time in nature and engaging in outdoor activities can have a calming effect on the mind and body. Nature walks, hiking, gardening, and other outdoor pursuits can reduce stress levels, improve mood, and boost immune function.

5. **Social Support and Connection**: Maintaining social connections and seeking support from friends, family, or support groups can provide emotional comfort and buffer against the negative effects of stress. Building strong social networks can enhance resilience and promote overall well-being.

Sleep Improvement Strategies

Quality sleep is essential for immune function, cognitive function, and overall health. Dr. Barbara recommends the following sleep improvement strategies to support immune support:

1. **Establishing a Sleep Routine**: Consistency is key for optimizing sleep quality and quantity. Establishing a regular sleep schedule, with consistent bedtimes and wake-up times, helps regulate the body's internal clock and improve sleep-wake cycles.

2. **Creating a Relaxing Bedtime Routine**: Engaging in relaxing activities before bedtime can help signal to the body that it's time to wind down and prepare for sleep. Activities such as reading, taking a warm bath, practicing relaxation techniques, or listening to calming music can promote relaxation and improve sleep quality.

3. **Optimizing Sleep Environment**: Creating a comfortable sleep environment is essential for promoting restful sleep. This includes keeping the bedroom dark, quiet, and cool, investing in a supportive mattress and pillows, and minimizing exposure to electronic devices and screens before bedtime.

4. **Limiting Stimulants and Alcohol**: Stimulants such as caffeine and nicotine can interfere with sleep quality and disrupt sleep patterns. Dr. Barbara recommends limiting caffeine

intake, especially in the afternoon and evening, and avoiding alcohol close to bedtime, as it can disrupt sleep architecture and lead to fragmented sleep.

5. **Managing Stress and Anxiety**: Stress and anxiety can interfere with sleep initiation and maintenance. Practicing stress reduction techniques, such as mindfulness meditation, deep breathing exercises, or progressive muscle relaxation, can help calm the mind and promote better sleep.

Regular Exercise

Regular physical activity is essential for supporting immune function, reducing inflammation, and promoting overall health and well-being. Dr. Barbara recommends the following exercise strategies to enhance immune support:

1. **Aerobic Exercise**: Aerobic exercise, such as walking, jogging, swimming, or cycling, increases heart rate and breathing rate, promoting cardiovascular health and improving circulation. Regular aerobic exercise can also reduce stress, boost mood, and enhance immune function.

2. **Strength Training**: Strength training, using weights, resistance bands, or body weight exercises, helps build muscle strength and endurance, improve bone density, and increase metabolic rate. Strength training exercises should

target major muscle groups and be performed at least two to three times per week.

3. **Flexibility and Balance Exercises**: Flexibility and balance exercises, such as yoga, Pilates, or stretching routines, improve joint mobility, enhance flexibility, and reduce the risk of injury. These exercises also promote relaxation, reduce muscle tension, and support overall well-being.

4. **Outdoor Activities**: Engaging in outdoor activities, such as hiking, gardening, or playing sports, provides additional benefits beyond physical exercise. Spending time outdoors exposes the body to natural sunlight, which helps regulate the sleep-wake cycle, boosts mood, and supports immune function.

5. **Mindful Movement Practices**: Mindful movement practices, such as tai chi, qigong, or mindful walking, combine gentle movements with focused attention and deep breathing to promote relaxation, reduce stress, and improve overall well-being.

Conclusion

Incorporating lifestyle modifications such as stress reduction, sleep improvement, and regular exercise is essential for supporting immune function and promoting overall health and well-being. Dr. Barbara's approach emphasizes holistic strategies that address the mind, body, and spirit to enhance immune support and resilience against infections. By adopting healthy lifestyle habits and incorporating stress reduction techniques, sleep improvement strategies, and regular exercise into daily routines, individuals can optimize immune function, reduce inflammation, and enhance quality of life.

CHAPTER SIX

Implementing Dr. Barbara's Protocol: Practical Steps for Incorporating Her Recommendations into Daily Life

Dr. Barbara's holistic approach to health and immune support encompasses a range of strategies, including nutrition, herbal remedies, lifestyle modifications, and stress reduction techniques. Implementing her protocol into daily life requires a commitment to prioritizing self-care and adopting healthy habits. Here are practical steps for incorporating Dr. Barbara's recommendations into daily routines:

1. Establish Clear Goals:

- Define specific health goals based on Dr. Barbara's recommendations. Whether it's improving immune function, reducing stress, or enhancing overall well-being, having clear goals will guide your efforts and keep you motivated.

2. Educate Yourself:

- Take the time to learn about Dr. Barbara's protocol and the rationale behind her recommendations. Understanding the science and principles behind each strategy will help you make informed decisions and stay committed to the protocol.

3. Consult with a Healthcare Professional:

- Before making any significant changes to your lifestyle or starting new supplements, consult with a healthcare professional, such as a doctor, nutritionist, or herbalist. They can provide personalized guidance based on your individual health needs and medical history.

4. Create a Wellness Plan:

- Develop a comprehensive wellness plan that incorporates Dr. Barbara's recommendations into your daily life. This plan should include dietary guidelines, herbal remedies, exercise routines, stress reduction techniques, and strategies for improving sleep quality.

5. Prioritize Nutrition:

- Follow Dr. Barbara's dietary recommendations by incorporating nutrient-dense foods into your meals. Focus on fruits, vegetables, whole grains, lean proteins, and healthy fats to provide essential vitamins, minerals, and antioxidants for immune support.

6. Incorporate Herbal Remedies:

- Integrate immune-boosting herbs and supplements recommended by Dr. Barbara into your daily routine. Whether it's echinacea, astragalus, elderberry, or medicinal mushrooms, take these herbs consistently as directed to support immune function.

7. Practice Stress Reduction Techniques:

- Dedicate time each day to practice stress reduction techniques such as mindfulness meditation, deep breathing exercises, yoga, or tai chi. Set aside a quiet space where you can relax and unwind, even if it's just for a few minutes each day.

8. Prioritize Sleep:

- Improve your sleep hygiene by creating a calming bedtime routine and optimizing your sleep environment. Establish a regular sleep schedule, limit screen time before bed, and create a comfortable sleep environment conducive to restorative sleep.

9. Incorporate Regular Exercise:

- Make physical activity a priority by incorporating regular exercise into your daily routine. Choose activities you enjoy, whether it's walking, jogging, cycling, or yoga, and aim for at least 30 minutes of moderate-intensity exercise most days of the week.

10. Monitor Progress and Adjust as Needed:

- Keep track of your progress towards your health goals and make adjustments to your wellness plan as needed. Listen to your body and pay attention to how different strategies impact your health and well-being.

11. Stay Consistent and Persistent:

- Incorporating Dr. Barbara's protocol into daily life requires consistency and persistence. Stay committed to your wellness plan, even on days when it feels challenging, and remember that small, consistent actions over time can lead to significant improvements in health and well-being.

12. Seek Support and Accountability:

- Surround yourself with supportive individuals who can encourage and motivate you on your wellness journey. Consider joining a support group, working with a health coach, or partnering with a friend or family member who shares your health goals.

By implementing Dr. Barbara's protocol into your daily life and committing to prioritizing self-care and healthy habits, you can enhance immune support, reduce stress, and improve overall well-being. Remember that health is a journey, and every small step you take towards better health matters.

CHAPTER SEVEN

Healing Testimonials: Inspiring Stories of Individuals Who Have Experienced Improvements in HIV/AIDS Symptoms with Dr. Barbara's Approach

Dr. Barbara's holistic approach to managing HIV/AIDS has transformed the lives of many individuals, empowering them to take charge of their health and well-being. Through a combination of nutrition, herbal remedies, lifestyle modifications, and stress reduction techniques, Dr. Barbara's protocol has helped individuals living with HIV/AIDS experience improvements in symptoms, immune function, and overall quality of life. Here are some inspiring testimonials from individuals who have benefited from Dr. Barbara's approach:

1. Mark's Story: Reclaiming Health and Vitality

- Mark was diagnosed with HIV/AIDS several years ago and struggled with managing his symptoms and maintaining his health. After learning about Dr. Barbara's holistic approach, Mark decided to incorporate her recommendations into his daily life. By following a nutrient-rich diet, incorporating immune-boosting herbs and supplements, practicing stress reduction techniques, and prioritizing self-care, Mark experienced significant improvements in his energy levels, immune function, and overall well-being. Today, Mark feels more empowered and resilient in managing his HIV/AIDS, reclaiming his health and vitality with Dr. Barbara's guidance.

2. Sarah's Journey: Thriving Despite the Challenges

- Sarah was diagnosed with HIV/AIDS during her pregnancy and faced numerous challenges in managing her health while caring for her newborn child. Despite the obstacles she encountered, Sarah remained determined to prioritize her well-being and explore alternative approaches to managing her condition. With Dr. Barbara's guidance, Sarah implemented dietary changes, herbal remedies, and stress reduction techniques into her daily routine. Over time, Sarah noticed improvements in her immune function, energy levels, and overall health, allowing her to thrive despite the challenges of living with HIV/AIDS. Today, Sarah serves as an inspiration to others, demonstrating that with dedication and support, it's possible to live a fulfilling and healthy life with HIV/AIDS.

3. Carlos' Transformation: Overcoming Adversity with Resilience

- Carlos was diagnosed with HIV/AIDS at a young age and faced numerous health challenges as a result of his condition. Despite the setbacks he encountered, Carlos remained determined to improve his health and quality of life. With the guidance of Dr. Barbara, Carlos embarked on a holistic healing journey that encompassed dietary changes, herbal remedies, stress reduction techniques, and regular exercise. Through perseverance and resilience, Carlos experienced remarkable improvements in his immune function, symptom management, and overall well-being. Today, Carlos serves as a beacon of hope for others living with HIV/AIDS, demonstrating that with the right support and mindset, it's possible to overcome adversity and thrive.

4. Maria's Testimony: Embracing Wellness and Empowerment

- Maria was diagnosed with HIV/AIDS and initially felt overwhelmed and uncertain about her future. However, with the guidance of Dr. Barbara, Maria embarked on a journey of self-discovery and empowerment. Through dietary changes, herbal remedies, stress reduction techniques, and lifestyle modifications, Maria experienced profound improvements in her health and well-being. She regained her energy, strengthened her immune system, and embraced a sense of wellness and vitality she never thought possible. Today, Maria lives her life with purpose and passion, serving as a testament to the transformative power of holistic healing and self-care.

These inspiring testimonials demonstrate the profound impact of Dr. Barbara's holistic approach to managing HIV/AIDS. By empowering individuals to take charge of their health and well-being through nutrition, herbal remedies, lifestyle modifications, and stress reduction techniques, Dr. Barbara's protocol offers hope and healing to those living with HIV/AIDS. Through dedication, perseverance, and support, individuals can experience improvements in symptoms, immune function, and overall quality of life, reclaiming their health and vitality in the face of adversity.

CHAPTER EIGHT

Monitoring HIV/AIDS Progression: Understanding How to Track Viral Load and CD4 Counts

Monitoring HIV/AIDS progression is essential for assessing disease status, guiding treatment decisions, and optimizing patient care. Two key markers used to monitor HIV/AIDS progression are viral load and CD4 counts. Understanding how to track these markers provides valuable insight into the immune status and viral activity in individuals living with HIV/AIDS.

Viral Load

Viral load refers to the amount of HIV RNA present in a blood sample and serves as a measure of the level of viral replication in the body. Monitoring viral load is crucial for assessing the effectiveness of antiretroviral therapy (ART) and guiding treatment decisions. Here's how viral load testing works:

1. **Testing Procedure**: Viral load testing involves collecting a blood sample from the individual and measuring the amount of HIV RNA present in the sample using a technique called polymerase chain reaction (PCR). This highly sensitive test can detect even small amounts of viral RNA in the blood.

2. **Interpretation**: Viral load results are reported as the number of copies of HIV RNA per milliliter of blood (copies/mL). A

low viral load indicates that HIV replication is suppressed, while a high viral load suggests active viral replication and a greater risk of disease progression and transmission.

3. **Monitoring**: Viral load testing is typically performed at regular intervals, such as every three to six months, to assess the effectiveness of ART and monitor disease progression over time. Consistently undetectable viral load levels (<50 copies/mL) are associated with improved health outcomes and a reduced risk of transmission.

4. **Treatment Response**: Viral load testing is used to assess the response to antiretroviral therapy (ART). A decrease in viral load after starting ART indicates that the treatment is working effectively to suppress viral replication. Consistently low or undetectable viral load levels are the goal of HIV treatment and are associated with better long-term outcomes.

CD4 Counts

CD4 counts refer to the number of CD4 T cells, a type of white blood cell, present in a blood sample and serve as a measure of immune function. Monitoring CD4 counts is essential for assessing immune status, guiding treatment decisions, and predicting the risk of opportunistic infections. Here's how CD4 count testing works:

1. **Testing Procedure**: CD4 count testing involves collecting a blood sample from the individual and measuring the number of CD4 T cells present in the sample using flow cytometry. This technique allows for the enumeration of specific cell populations based on their surface markers.

2. **Interpretation**: CD4 counts are reported as the number of CD4 T cells per cubic millimeter of blood (cells/mm³). Higher CD4 counts indicate a stronger immune system, while lower CD4 counts suggest immune suppression and an increased risk of opportunistic infections.

3. **Monitoring**: CD4 count testing is typically performed at regular intervals, such as every three to six months, to assess immune function and monitor disease progression over time. Changes in CD4 counts can indicate changes in immune status and may prompt adjustments to treatment strategies.

4. **Treatment Thresholds**: CD4 count thresholds are used to guide treatment decisions in individuals with HIV/AIDS. Historically, treatment initiation was recommended when CD4 counts fell below a certain threshold (e.g., <350 cells/mm³). However, current guidelines recommend initiating ART regardless of CD4 count to achieve viral suppression and prevent disease progression.

Conclusion

Monitoring HIV/AIDS progression involves tracking viral load and CD4 counts to assess viral activity and immune function. Viral load testing measures the amount of HIV RNA in the blood and helps assess the effectiveness of antiretroviral therapy. CD4 count testing measures the number of CD4 T cells in the blood and provides valuable information about immune function and the risk of opportunistic infections. By monitoring these markers regularly and adjusting treatment strategies as needed, healthcare providers can optimize patient care and improve long-term outcomes for individuals living with HIV/AIDS.

CHAPTER NINE

Holistic Wellness Practices: Nurturing Mind, Body, and Spirit for Comprehensive Immune Support

Holistic wellness practices encompass a wide range of approaches that address the interconnectedness of mind, body, and spirit to promote overall health and well-being. By nurturing all aspects of health, holistic practices provide comprehensive support for immune function, stress reduction, and overall vitality. Here are some holistic wellness practices that can contribute to comprehensive immune support:

1. Mindfulness Meditation and Stress Reduction Techniques:

- Mindfulness meditation involves bringing attention to the present moment with openness and acceptance, which can help reduce stress, anxiety, and negative emotions. Other stress reduction techniques, such as deep breathing exercises, progressive muscle relaxation, and guided imagery, promote relaxation and support immune function by reducing the production of stress hormones.

2. Nutrient-Rich Diet and Herbal Supplements:

- A nutrient-rich diet that includes a variety of fruits, vegetables, whole grains, lean proteins, and healthy fats provides essential vitamins, minerals, antioxidants, and phytonutrients necessary for immune function. Herbal supplements, such as echinacea, astragalus, elderberry, and medicinal mushrooms, offer additional immune-boosting support and can be incorporated into daily wellness routines.

3. Regular Exercise and Physical Activity:

- Regular exercise and physical activity support immune function by promoting circulation, reducing inflammation, and enhancing overall health. Engaging in activities such as walking, jogging, swimming, or yoga not only strengthens the body but also boosts mood, reduces stress, and supports immune resilience.

4. Quality Sleep and Restorative Practices:

- Quality sleep is essential for immune function, cognitive function, and overall well-being. Prioritizing sleep hygiene, establishing a relaxing bedtime routine, and creating a comfortable sleep environment can promote restorative sleep and enhance immune support. Restorative practices such as meditation, gentle yoga, or tai chi can also help reduce stress and promote relaxation for improved sleep quality.

5. Connection and Social Support:

- Maintaining meaningful connections with others and seeking social support are vital aspects of holistic wellness. Strong social networks provide emotional comfort, reduce feelings of loneliness and isolation, and promote resilience in the face of stress. Whether through spending time with loved ones, participating in community activities, or joining support groups, fostering connections contributes to overall well-being and immune support.

6. Nature Therapy and Outdoor Activities:

- Spending time in nature, also known as nature therapy or ecotherapy, has been shown to have numerous health benefits, including stress reduction, improved mood, and enhanced immune function. Engaging in outdoor activities such as hiking, gardening, or simply taking a walk in nature can provide opportunities for relaxation, reflection, and connection with the natural world.

7. Creative Expression and Self-Care Practices:

- Engaging in creative expression, whether through art, music, writing, or other forms of self-expression, can be therapeutic and nourishing for the mind, body, and spirit. Practicing self-care activities such as journaling, taking a bath, or indulging in a hobby can help reduce stress, promote relaxation, and support overall well-being.

8. Mind-Body Practices and Energy Healing Modalities:

- Mind-body practices such as yoga, tai chi, qigong, and acupuncture integrate movement, breathwork, and mindfulness to promote balance and harmony within the body. Energy healing modalities such as Reiki, acupuncture, or energy work focus on restoring the flow of energy and promoting healing on a holistic level, supporting immune function and overall vitality.

By incorporating these holistic wellness practices into daily life, individuals can nurture their mind, body, and spirit for comprehensive immune support. By addressing the interconnectedness of all aspects of health, holistic approaches promote resilience, vitality, and well-being, supporting overall immune function and enhancing quality of life.

CHAPTER TEN

Beyond HIV/AIDS: Sustaining Overall Health and Wellness Through Long-Term Preventive Practices and Dietary Habits

While managing HIV/AIDS is a critical aspect of maintaining health, sustaining overall well-being requires a long-term commitment to preventive practices and healthy dietary habits. By adopting a proactive approach to health and wellness, individuals can optimize immune function, reduce the risk of chronic diseases, and enhance quality of life. Here are some key preventive practices and dietary habits to promote long-term health and wellness:

1. Regular Exercise and Physical Activity:

- Incorporating regular exercise and physical activity into daily routines is essential for maintaining cardiovascular health, strengthening the immune system, and promoting overall well-being. Aim for a combination of aerobic exercise, strength training, and flexibility exercises to support optimal health and vitality.

2. Nutrient-Rich Diet:

- Consuming a nutrient-rich diet that emphasizes whole foods such as fruits, vegetables, whole grains, lean proteins, and healthy fats provides essential vitamins, minerals, antioxidants, and phytonutrients necessary for immune function and overall health. Limit processed foods, sugary beverages, and excessive salt intake, and prioritize nutrient-dense foods to fuel your body and support long-term wellness.

3. Adequate Hydration:

- Staying hydrated is crucial for maintaining proper bodily functions, supporting immune function, and promoting overall health. Aim to drink plenty of water throughout the day and limit the consumption of sugary drinks and caffeinated beverages.

4. Stress Reduction Techniques:

- Chronic stress can weaken the immune system, increase inflammation, and contribute to the development of chronic diseases. Incorporate stress reduction techniques such as mindfulness meditation, deep breathing exercises, yoga, or tai chi into your daily routine to promote relaxation, resilience, and overall well-being.

5. Quality Sleep:

- Prioritize quality sleep by establishing a consistent sleep schedule, creating a relaxing bedtime routine, and optimizing your sleep environment. Aim for seven to nine hours of restorative sleep each night to support immune function, cognitive function, and overall health.

6. Regular Health Screenings and Check-Ups:

- Schedule regular health screenings and check-ups with your healthcare provider to monitor key health indicators, detect potential health issues early, and make informed decisions about preventive care and treatment options.

7. Maintain a Healthy Weight:

- Maintaining a healthy weight through balanced nutrition and regular exercise is important for reducing the risk of chronic diseases such as diabetes, heart disease, and certain cancers. Aim for a balanced diet and engage in regular physical activity to support weight management and overall health.

8. Limit Alcohol and Avoid Tobacco:

- Limit alcohol consumption and avoid tobacco use to reduce the risk of chronic diseases and promote overall health. Excessive alcohol consumption and tobacco use are associated with an increased risk of cardiovascular disease, cancer, and other health conditions.

9. Foster Social Connections:

- Cultivate meaningful social connections and maintain a strong support network to promote emotional well-being, reduce feelings of loneliness and isolation, and enhance overall quality of life.

10. Practice Gratitude and Positive Thinking:

- Cultivate an attitude of gratitude and positive thinking to promote resilience, enhance mental health, and improve overall well-being. Focus on the present moment, practice self-compassion, and find joy in everyday experiences to nurture your mind, body, and spirit.

By adopting these preventive practices and healthy dietary habits, individuals can sustain overall health and wellness for the long term. By prioritizing proactive health behaviors and making informed lifestyle choices, individuals can optimize immune function, reduce the risk of chronic diseases, and enhance quality of life, supporting long-term well-being and vitality.

Valerian:

Definition: Valerian, scientifically known as Valeriana officinalis, is a perennial flowering plant native to Europe and Asia. It has been used for centuries in traditional medicine for its potential calming and sedative effects.

Ingredients: Valerian root contains several bioactive compounds, including valerenic acid, valepotriates, and volatile oils. These compounds are believed to contribute to the herb's medicinal properties, including its potential as a sedative, anxiolytic, and sleep aid.

How to Prepare: Valerian root is typically prepared and consumed as an herbal tea, tincture, or capsule. To make tea, dried valerian root is steeped in hot water for several minutes before being strained and consumed. Tinctures are prepared by steeping the root in alcohol or vinegar to extract its active compounds.

Dosage: The appropriate dosage of valerian can vary depending on factors such as age, health status, and the specific preparation being used. It's important to follow the recommended dosage on the product label or consult with a qualified herbalist or healthcare professional for personalized guidance.

How to Use: Valerian tea, tincture, or capsules are typically taken orally. It's often consumed in the evening as a sleep aid or during times of stress or anxiety. It's important to use valerian products as directed and to discontinue use if any adverse effects occur.

Side Effects: Valerian is generally considered safe for most people when used in moderate amounts. However, some individuals may experience mild side effects such as drowsiness, headache, or gastrointestinal upset. It may also interact with certain medications or have adverse effects in individuals with certain health conditions. It's important to use valerian under the guidance of a healthcare professional and to discontinue use if any adverse effects occur.

BONUS: SOME HERBAL REMEDIES TO KNOW

Wild Cherry Bark:

Definition: Wild cherry bark, scientifically known as Prunus serotina, is the bark obtained from the black cherry tree native to North America. It has been used traditionally in Native American and folk medicine for its potential health benefits, particularly for respiratory and digestive issues.

Ingredients: Wild cherry bark contains various bioactive compounds, including cyanogenic glycosides (such as prunasin and amygdalin), flavonoids, and phenolic acids. These compounds are believed to contribute to the herb's medicinal properties, including its potential as an expectorant, cough suppressant, and mild sedative.

How to Prepare: Wild cherry bark is typically prepared and consumed as an herbal tea, decoction, or syrup. To make tea, dried wild cherry bark is steeped in hot water for several minutes before being strained and consumed. Decoctions involve boiling the bark in water to extract its active compounds, while syrups are made by simmering the bark with sugar or honey to create a thick, sweet liquid.

Dosage: The appropriate dosage of wild cherry bark can vary depending on factors such as age, health status, and the specific preparation being used. It's important to follow the recommended dosage on the product label or consult with a qualified herbalist or healthcare professional for personalized guidance.

How to Use: Wild cherry bark tea, decoction, or syrup is typically taken orally. It's often consumed to soothe coughs, sore throats, and other respiratory symptoms. It's important to use wild cherry bark products as directed and to discontinue use if any adverse effects occur.

Side Effects: Wild cherry bark is generally considered safe for most people when used in moderate amounts. However, it contains cyanogenic glycosides, which can release cyanide in the body when metabolized. While the risk of cyanide poisoning from consuming wild cherry bark is low when used appropriately, excessive intake or prolonged use may lead to adverse effects. It's important to use wild cherry bark under the guidance of a healthcare professional and to discontinue use if any adverse effects occur.

Yellowdock:

Definition: Yellowdock, scientifically known as Rumex crispus, is a perennial flowering plant native to Europe and western Asia but is also found in North America. It has a long history of use in traditional medicine, particularly among Indigenous peoples, for its potential health benefits.

Ingredients: Yellowdock root contains various bioactive compounds, including anthraquinone glycosides (such as emodin and chrysophanol), tannins, and vitamins (including vitamin A and vitamin C). These compounds are believed to contribute to the herb's medicinal properties, including its potential as a laxative, blood cleanser, and liver tonic.

How to Prepare: Yellowdock root is typically prepared and consumed as an herbal tea, tincture, or capsule. To make tea, dried yellowdock root is steeped in hot water for several minutes before being strained and consumed. Tinctures are prepared by steeping the root in alcohol or vinegar to extract its active compounds.

Dosage: The appropriate dosage of yellowdock can vary depending on factors such as age, health status, and the specific preparation being used. It's important to follow the recommended dosage on the product label or consult with a qualified herbalist or healthcare professional for personalized guidance.

How to Use: Yellowdock tea, tincture, or capsules are typically taken orally. It's often consumed to support digestion, promote bowel regularity, and cleanse the blood. It's important to use yellowdock products as directed and to discontinue use if any adverse effects occur.

Side Effects: Yellowdock is generally considered safe for most people when used in moderate amounts. However, some individuals may experience mild side effects such as gastrointestinal upset or allergic reactions. It may also interact with certain medications or have adverse effects in individuals with certain health conditions. It's important to use yellowdock under the guidance of a healthcare professional and to discontinue use if any adverse effects occur.

Yellowdock Root:

Definition: Yellowdock root, scientifically known as Rumex crispus, is the root of a perennial flowering plant native to Europe and western Asia, also found in North America. It has a long history of use in traditional medicine, particularly among Indigenous peoples, for its potential health benefits.

Ingredients: Yellowdock root contains various bioactive compounds, including anthraquinone glycosides (such as emodin and chrysophanol), tannins, and vitamins (including vitamin A and vitamin C). These compounds are believed to contribute to the herb's medicinal properties, including its potential as a laxative, blood cleanser, and liver tonic.

How to Prepare: Yellowdock root is typically prepared and consumed as an herbal tea, tincture, or capsule. To make tea, dried yellowdock root is steeped in hot water for several minutes before being strained and consumed. Tinctures are prepared by steeping the root in alcohol or vinegar to extract its active compounds.

Dosage: The appropriate dosage of yellowdock root can vary depending on factors such as age, health status, and the specific preparation being used. It's important to follow the recommended dosage on the product label or consult with a qualified herbalist or healthcare professional for personalized guidance.

How to Use: Yellowdock root tea, tincture, or capsules are typically taken orally. It's often consumed to support digestion, promote bowel regularity, and cleanse the blood. It's important to use yellowdock root products as directed and to discontinue use if any adverse effects occur.

Side Effects: Yellowdock root is generally considered safe for most people when used in moderate amounts. However, some individuals may experience mild side effects such as gastrointestinal upset or allergic reactions. It may also interact with certain medications or have adverse effects in individuals with certain health conditions. It's important to use yellowdock root under the guidance of a healthcare professional and to discontinue use if any adverse effects occur.

Agrimony:

Definition: Agrimony, scientifically known as Agrimonia eupatoria, is a perennial herbaceous plant native to Europe, Asia, and North America. It has a long history of use in traditional medicine, particularly in European folk medicine, for its potential health benefits.

Ingredients: Agrimony contains various bioactive compounds, including tannins, flavonoids, phenolic acids, and volatile oils. These compounds are believed to contribute to the herb's medicinal properties, including its potential as an astringent, anti-inflammatory, and digestive aid.

How to Prepare: Agrimony is typically prepared and consumed as an herbal tea, tincture, or poultice. To make tea, dried agrimony leaves and flowers are steeped in hot water for several minutes before being strained and consumed. Tinctures are prepared by steeping the herb in alcohol or vinegar to extract its active compounds.

Dosage: The appropriate dosage of agrimony can vary depending on factors such as age, health status, and the specific preparation being used. It's important to follow the recommended dosage on the product label or consult with a qualified herbalist or healthcare professional for personalized guidance.

How to Use: Agrimony tea, tincture, or poultice is typically taken orally or applied topically. It's often consumed to soothe gastrointestinal issues, such as indigestion and diarrhea, or used externally to treat skin conditions.

Side Effects: Agrimony is generally considered safe for most people when used in moderate amounts. However, some individuals may experience allergic reactions or gastrointestinal upset. It may also interact with certain medications or have adverse effects in individuals with certain health conditions. It's important to use agrimony under the guidance of a healthcare professional and to discontinue use if any adverse effects occur.

Alfalfa:

Definition: Alfalfa, scientifically known as Medicago sativa, is a flowering plant in the pea family native to Asia but cultivated worldwide. It's primarily grown as fodder for livestock, but it has also been used in traditional medicine for its potential health benefits.

Ingredients: Alfalfa contains various bioactive compounds, including vitamins (such as vitamin A, vitamin C, and vitamin K), minerals (including calcium, magnesium, and potassium), amino acids, and phytoestrogens. These compounds are believed to contribute to the herb's medicinal properties, including its potential as a nutritive tonic, diuretic, and hormone balancer.

How to Prepare: Alfalfa is typically consumed as sprouts, herbal tea, or in supplement form (such as capsules or tablets). To make tea, dried alfalfa leaves are steeped in hot water for several minutes before being strained and consumed.

Dosage: The appropriate dosage of alfalfa can vary depending on factors such as age, health status, and the specific preparation being used. It's important to follow the recommended dosage on the product label or consult with a qualified herbalist or healthcare professional for personalized guidance.

How to Use: Alfalfa sprouts, tea, or supplements are typically taken orally. It's often consumed as a dietary supplement to support overall health and well-being, as well as to promote kidney health and hormone balance.

Side Effects: Alfalfa is generally considered safe for most people when consumed in moderate amounts. However, some individuals may experience allergic reactions or digestive upset. It may also interact with certain medications or have adverse effects in individuals with certain health conditions, such as autoimmune diseases or hormone-sensitive conditions. Pregnant or breastfeeding individuals should consult with a healthcare professional before using alfalfa supplements. It's important to use alfalfa under the guidance of a healthcare professional and to discontinue use if any adverse effects occur.

Ashwagandha:

Definition: Ashwagandha, scientifically known as Withaniasomnifera, is a small shrub native to India, the Middle East, and parts of Africa. It has a long history of use in Ayurvedic medicine for its potential health benefits, particularly for its adaptogenic properties.

Ingredients: Ashwagandha root contains various bioactive compounds, including alkaloids (such as withanolides), steroidal lactones, and flavonoids. These compounds are believed to contribute to the herb's medicinal properties, including its potential as an adaptogen, anti-inflammatory, and immune-modulating agent.

How to Prepare: Ashwagandha is typically consumed as a powdered root, herbal tea, tincture, or in supplement form (such as capsules or tablets). To make tea, dried ashwagandha root is steeped in hot water for several minutes before being strained and consumed.

Dosage: The appropriate dosage of ashwagandha can vary depending on factors such as age, health status, and the specific preparation being used. It's important to follow the recommended dosage on the product label or consult with a qualified herbalist or healthcare professional for personalized guidance.

How to Use: Ashwagandha powder, tea, tincture, or supplements are typically taken orally. It's often consumed to support stress management, promote relaxation, and boost overall vitality and well-being.

Side Effects: Ashwagandha is generally considered safe for most people when used in moderate amounts. However, some individuals may experience mild side effects such as gastrointestinal upset or drowsiness. It may also interact with certain medications or have adverse effects in individuals with certain health conditions, such as autoimmune diseases or thyroid disorders. Pregnant or breastfeeding individuals should consult with a healthcare professional before using ashwagandha supplements. It's important to use ashwagandha under the guidance of a healthcare professional and to discontinue use if any adverse effects occur.

Astragalus:

Definition: Astragalus, scientifically known as Astragalus membranaceus, is a flowering plant native to China and Mongolia but also found in other parts of Asia. It has been used for centuries in traditional Chinese medicine for its potential health benefits, particularly for its immune-enhancing properties.

Ingredients: Astragalus root contains various bioactive compounds, including polysaccharides, saponins (such as astragalosides), flavonoids, and amino acids. These compounds are believed to contribute to the herb's medicinal properties, including its potential as an adaptogen, immunomodulator, and anti-inflammatory agent.

How to Prepare: Astragalus is typically consumed as a powdered root, herbal tea, tincture, or in supplement form (such as capsules or tablets). To make tea, dried astragalus root slices are simmered in water for several minutes before being strained and consumed.

Dosage: The appropriate dosage of astragalus can vary depending on factors such as age, health status, and the specific preparation being used. It's important to follow the recommended dosage on the product label or consult with a qualified herbalist or healthcare professional for personalized guidance.

How to Use: Astragalus powder, tea, tincture, or supplements are typically taken orally. It's often consumed to support immune function, promote vitality, and enhance overall well-being.

Side Effects: Astragalus is generally considered safe for most people when used in moderate amounts. However, some individuals may experience mild side effects such as gastrointestinal upset or allergic reactions. It may also interact with certain medications or have adverse effects in individuals with certain health conditions, such as autoimmune diseases or diabetes. Pregnant or breastfeeding individuals should consult with a healthcare professional before using astragalus supplements. It's important to use astragalus under the guidance of a healthcare professional and to discontinue use if any adverse effects occur.

Black Cohosh:

Definition: Black cohosh, scientifically known as Actaea racemosa (formerly Cimicifuga racemosa), is a perennial herb native to North America. It has a long history of use in traditional Native American medicine and later in folk medicine for its potential health benefits, particularly for women's health.

Ingredients: Black cohosh root contains various bioactive compounds, including triterpene glycosides (such as actein and cimicifugoside), phenolic acids, and flavonoids. These compounds are believed to contribute to the herb's medicinal properties, including its potential as a hormone-balancing agent and its ability to relieve menopausal symptoms.

How to Prepare: Black cohosh is typically consumed as a powdered root, herbal tea, tincture, or in supplement form (such as capsules or tablets). To make tea, dried black cohosh root is steeped in hot water for several minutes before being strained and consumed.

Dosage: The appropriate dosage of black cohosh can vary depending on factors such as age, health status, and the specific preparation being used. It's important to follow the recommended dosage on the product label or consult with a qualified herbalist or healthcare professional for personalized guidance.

How to Use: Black cohosh powder, tea, tincture, or supplements are typically taken orally. It's often used by women to support hormonal balance, relieve menopausal symptoms such as hot flashes and night sweats, and promote overall well-being.

Side Effects: Black cohosh is generally considered safe for most people when used in moderate amounts. However, some individuals may experience mild side effects such as gastrointestinal upset or allergic reactions. It may also interact with certain medications or have adverse effects in individuals with certain health conditions, such as liver disease or hormone-sensitive conditions. Pregnant or breastfeeding individuals should consult with a healthcare professional before using black cohosh supplements. It's important to use black cohosh under the guidance of a healthcare professional and to discontinue use if any adverse effects occur.

Blessed Thistle:

Definition: Blessed thistle, scientifically known as Cnicusbenedictus, is an annual or biennial herb native to the Mediterranean region but also found in other parts of Europe, Asia, and North Africa. It has been used historically in traditional medicine for its potential health benefits, particularly for digestive and liver health.

Ingredients: Blessed thistle contains various bioactive compounds, including sesquiterpene lactones (such as cnicin), flavonoids, tannins, and essential oils. These compounds are believed to contribute to the herb's medicinal properties, including its potential as a digestive tonic, appetite stimulant, and liver tonic.

How to Prepare: Blessed thistle is typically consumed as an herbal tea, tincture, or in supplement form (such as capsules or tablets). To make tea, dried blessed thistle leaves and flowers are steeped in hot water for several minutes before being strained and consumed.

Dosage: The appropriate dosage of blessed thistle can vary depending on factors such as age, health status, and the specific preparation being used. It's important to follow the recommended dosage on the product label or consult with a qualified herbalist or healthcare professional for personalized guidance.

How to Use: Blessed thistle tea, tincture, or supplements are typically taken orally. It's often used to support digestion, stimulate appetite, and promote liver health.

Side Effects: Blessed thistle is generally considered safe for most people when used in moderate amounts. However, some individuals may experience mild side effects such as gastrointestinal upset or allergic reactions. It may also interact with certain medications or have adverse effects in individuals with certain health conditions, such as hormone-sensitive conditions or bleeding disorders. Pregnant or breastfeeding individuals should consult with a healthcare professional before using blessed thistle supplements. It's important to use blessed thistle under the guidance of a healthcare professional and to discontinue use if any adverse effects occur.

Cat's Claw:

Definition: Cat's claw, scientifically known as Uncaria tomentosa, is a woody vine native to the Amazon rainforest and other parts of Central and South America. It has been used for centuries in traditional medicine by indigenous peoples for its potential health benefits.

Ingredients: Cat's claw contains various bioactive compounds, including alkaloids (such as oxindole alkaloids and quinovic acid glycosides), polyphenols, and other phytochemicals. These compounds are believed to contribute to the herb's medicinal properties, including its potential as an immune enhancer, anti-inflammatory, and antioxidant.

How to Prepare: Cat's claw is typically consumed as an herbal tea, tincture, or in supplement form (such as capsules or tablets). To make tea, dried cat's claw bark or leaves are steeped in hot water for several minutes before being strained and consumed.

Dosage: The appropriate dosage of cat's claw can vary depending on factors such as age, health status, and the specific preparation being used. It's important to follow the recommended dosage on the product label or consult with a qualified herbalist or healthcare professional for personalized guidance.

How to Use: Cat's claw tea, tincture, or supplements are typically taken orally. It's often used to support immune function, reduce inflammation, and promote overall well-being.

Side Effects: Cat's claw is generally considered safe for most people when used in moderate amounts. However, some individuals may experience mild side effects such as gastrointestinal upset or allergic reactions. It may also interact with certain medications or have adverse effects in individuals with certain health conditions, such as autoimmune diseases or bleeding disorders. Pregnant or breastfeeding individuals should consult with a healthcare professional before using cat's claw supplements. It's important to use cat's claw under the guidance of a healthcare professional and to discontinue use if any adverse effects occur.

Chickweed:

Definition: Chickweed, scientifically known as Stellaria media, is an annual herbaceous plant native to Europe but naturalized in many other parts of the world. It's often considered a common weed but has been used historically in traditional medicine for its potential health benefits.

Ingredients: Chickweed contains various bioactive compounds, including flavonoids, saponins, mucilage, and vitamins (such as vitamin C). These compounds are believed to contribute to the herb's medicinal properties, including its potential as a demulcent, anti-inflammatory, and mild diuretic.

How to Prepare: Chickweed is typically consumed as an herbal tea, infusion, or in fresh salads. To make tea, dried chickweed leaves and flowers are steeped in hot water for several minutes before being strained and consumed. It can also be used topically as a poultice or infused oil for skin conditions.

Dosage: The appropriate dosage of chickweed can vary depending on factors such as age, health status, and the specific preparation being used. It's important to follow the recommended dosage on the product label or consult with a qualified herbalist or healthcare professional for personalized guidance.

How to Use: Chickweed tea, infusion, or fresh leaves are typically taken orally. It's often used to soothe inflammation, support digestion, and promote overall well-being. Topically, chickweed can be applied to the skin to alleviate itching, irritation, or minor wounds.

Side Effects: Chickweed is generally considered safe for most people when consumed in moderate amounts. However, some individuals may experience allergic reactions or gastrointestinal upset. It may also interact with certain medications or have adverse effects in individuals with certain health conditions. Pregnant or breastfeeding individuals should consult with a healthcare professional before using chickweed supplements. It's important to use chickweed under the guidance of a healthcare professional and to discontinue use if any adverse effects occur.

Cleavers:

Definition: Cleavers, scientifically known as Galium aparine, is a herbaceous annual plant native to Europe, North America, Asia, and Australia. It has a long history of use in traditional medicine for its potential health benefits.

Ingredients: Cleavers contains various bioactive compounds, including iridoid glycosides, flavonoids, tannins, and mucilage. These compounds are believed to contribute to the herb's medicinal properties, including its potential as a diuretic, lymphatic tonic, and mild astringent.

How to Prepare: Cleavers is typically consumed as an herbal tea, infusion, or in fresh salads. To make tea, dried cleavers leaves and stems are steeped in hot water for several minutes before being strained and consumed. It can also be used topically as a poultice or infused oil for skin conditions.

Dosage: The appropriate dosage of cleavers can vary depending on factors such as age, health status, and the specific preparation being used. It's important to follow the recommended dosage on the product label or consult with a qualified herbalist or healthcare professional for personalized guidance.

How to Use: Cleavers tea, infusion, or fresh leaves are typically taken orally. It's often used to support lymphatic drainage, promote urinary tract health, and soothe inflammation. Topically, cleavers can be applied to the skin to alleviate itching, irritation, or minor wounds.

Side Effects: Cleavers is generally considered safe for most people when consumed in moderate amounts. However, some individuals may experience allergic reactions or gastrointestinal upset. It may also interact with certain medications or have adverse effects in individuals with certain health conditions. Pregnant or breastfeeding individuals should consult with a healthcare professional before using cleavers supplements. It's important to use cleavers under the guidance of a healthcare professional and to discontinue use if any adverse effects occur.

Eucalyptus:

Definition: Eucalyptus refers to a genus of flowering trees and shrubs, primarily native to Australia but also found in other parts of the world. Eucalyptus essential oil, extracted from the leaves of certain species, has a long history of use in traditional medicine for its potential health benefits.

Ingredients: Eucalyptus essential oil contains various bioactive compounds, including eucalyptol (cineole), terpenes, and flavonoids. These compounds are believed to contribute to the oil's medicinal properties, including its potential as an expectorant, decongestant, antiseptic, and anti-inflammatory.

How to Prepare: Eucalyptus essential oil can be used in aromatherapy, diffused in the air, or diluted and applied topically to the skin. It can also be added to steam inhalations or chest rubs to help relieve respiratory symptoms.

Dosage: The appropriate dosage of eucalyptus essential oil can vary depending on factors such as age, health status, and the specific application being used. It's important to follow the recommended dosage on the product label or consult with a qualified aromatherapist or healthcare professional for personalized guidance.

How to Use: Eucalyptus essential oil can be used aromatically, topically, or internally, depending on the intended application. It's often used to alleviate respiratory congestion, soothe sore muscles, promote relaxation, and support overall well-being.

Side Effects: Eucalyptus essential oil is generally considered safe for most people when used appropriately. However, it can be toxic if ingested in large amounts and should not be applied directly to the skin without proper dilution. Some individuals may experience allergic reactions or respiratory irritation when exposed to eucalyptus oil. It's important to use eucalyptus oil with caution, especially around children and pets. Pregnant or breastfeeding individuals should consult with a healthcare professional before using eucalyptus oil. If any adverse effects occur, discontinue use and seek medical attention.

Feverfew:

Definition: Feverfew, scientifically known as Tanacetum parthenium, is a perennial herb native to Europe but also found in other parts of the world. It has a long history of use in traditional medicine, particularly in European folk medicine, for its potential health benefits.

Ingredients: Feverfew contains various bioactive compounds, including sesquiterpene lactones (such as parthenolide), flavonoids, and volatile oils. These compounds are believed to contribute to the herb's medicinal properties, including its potential as an anti-inflammatory, analgesic, and migraine prophylactic.

How to Prepare: Feverfew is typically consumed as an herbal tea, tincture, or in supplement form (such as capsules or tablets). To make tea, dried feverfew leaves and flowers are steeped in hot water for several minutes before being strained and consumed.

Dosage: The appropriate dosage of feverfew can vary depending on factors such as age, health status, and the specific preparation being used. It's important to follow the recommended dosage on the product label or consult with a qualified herbalist or healthcare professional for personalized guidance.

How to Use: Feverfew tea, tincture, or supplements are typically taken orally. It's often used to alleviate headaches, including migraines, and to support overall well-being.

Side Effects: Feverfew is generally considered safe for most people when used in moderate amounts. However, some individuals may experience mild side effects such as gastrointestinal upset or allergic reactions. It may also interact with certain medications or have adverse effects in individuals with certain health conditions, such as bleeding disorders or pregnancy. It's important to use feverfew under the guidance of a healthcare professional and to discontinue use if any adverse effects occur.

Ginseng:

Definition: Ginseng refers to several species of perennial plants belonging to the Panax genus, including Panax ginseng (Asian ginseng) and Panax quinquefolius (American ginseng). Ginseng has been used for centuries in traditional medicine, particularly in East Asia, for its potential health benefits.

Ingredients: Ginseng root contains various bioactive compounds, including ginsenosides, polysaccharides, and peptides. These compounds are believed to contribute to the herb's medicinal properties, including its potential as an adaptogen, immune enhancer, and cognitive booster.

How to Prepare: Ginseng is typically consumed as a powdered root, herbal tea, tincture, or in supplement form (such as capsules or tablets). To make tea, dried ginseng root slices are simmered in water for several minutes before being strained and consumed.

Dosage: The appropriate dosage of ginseng can vary depending on factors such as age, health status, and the specific preparation being used. It's important to follow the recommended dosage on the product label or consult with a qualified herbalist or healthcare professional for personalized guidance.

How to Use: Ginseng powder, tea, tincture, or supplements are typically taken orally. It's often used to support energy levels, enhance cognitive function, and promote overall well-being.

Side Effects: Ginseng is generally considered safe for most people when used in moderate amounts. However, some individuals may experience mild side effects such as insomnia, gastrointestinal upset, or headaches. It may also interact with certain medications or have adverse effects in individuals with certain health conditions, such as high blood pressure or diabetes. Pregnant or breastfeeding individuals should consult with a healthcare professional before using ginseng supplements. It's important to use ginseng under the guidance of a healthcare professional and to discontinue use if any adverse effects occur.

Bio Ferro Tonic:

Definition: Bio Ferro Tonic is a dietary supplement primarily composed of herbs and minerals. It's often marketed as a natural way to support overall health, particularly by promoting blood health and circulation.

Ingredients: Typical ingredients in Bio Ferro Tonic may include a blend of herbs such as burdock root, yellow dock root, sarsaparilla root, and cascara sagrada bark, along with minerals like iron and potassium phosphate.

How to Prepare: Bio Ferro Tonic usually comes in liquid form and is typically taken orally. It's important to follow the instructions on the product label for dosage and administration.

Dosage: The dosage can vary depending on the specific product and individual needs. It's crucial to consult with a healthcare professional or follow the recommended dosage on the product label to avoid potential side effects.

How to Use: Bio Ferro Tonic is often taken by adding the recommended dosage to water or juice and consuming it orally. It's important to shake the bottle well before use and store it according to the manufacturer's instructions.

Side Effects: While Bio Ferro Tonic is generally considered safe when used as directed, some individuals may experience side effects such as digestive discomfort, allergic reactions, or interactions with medications. It's essential to consult with a healthcare provider before starting any new supplement regimen, especially if you have underlying health conditions or are taking medications.

Blood Purifier:

Definition: Blood purifiers are herbal remedies or dietary supplements believed to cleanse or detoxify the blood, often promoting overall health and well-being. They are thought to support the body's natural detoxification processes and improve blood circulation.

Ingredients: Blood purifiers may contain a variety of herbs and botanical extracts known for their purported cleansing and detoxifying properties. Common ingredients include burdock root, red clover, dandelion root, and yellow dock root, among others.

How to Prepare: Blood purifiers are typically available in various forms, including capsules, tablets, powders, and liquid extracts. They are usually taken orally with water or juice, following the recommended dosage on the product label.

Dosage: The dosage of blood purifiers can vary depending on the specific product and individual needs. It's important to adhere to the recommended dosage on the product label or consult with a healthcare professional for personalized guidance.

How to Use: Blood purifiers are typically taken orally, either with water or mixed into beverages. They are often used as part of a detoxification regimen or to support overall health and vitality.

Side Effects: While blood purifiers are generally considered safe for most people when used as directed, some individuals may experience side effects such as digestive discomfort, allergic reactions, or interactions with medications. It's important to consult with a healthcare provider before starting any new supplement regimen, especially if you have underlying health conditions or are taking medications.

Blue Vervain:

Definition: Blue vervain, also known as Verbena hastata, is a perennial herb native to North America. It has been used in traditional medicine for centuries to treat various ailments, including anxiety, insomnia, and digestive issues.

Ingredients: Blue vervain contains several active compounds, including aucubin, verbenalin, and volatile oils. These compounds are believed to contribute to the herb's medicinal properties.

How to Prepare: Blue vervain is typically consumed as a tea or tincture. To make tea, dried blue vervain leaves and flowers are steeped in hot water for several minutes before being strained and consumed. Tinctures are prepared by steeping the herb in alcohol or vinegar to extract its active compounds.

Dosage: The appropriate dosage of blue vervain can vary depending on factors such as age, health status, and the specific preparation being used. It's important to follow the recommended dosage on the product label or consult with a qualified herbalist or healthcare professional for personalized guidance.

How to Use: Blue vervain tea or tincture is typically taken orally. It can be consumed on its own or mixed with honey or other herbal teas for added flavor.

Side Effects: While blue vervain is generally considered safe for most people when used in moderation, excessive intake may cause digestive upset or allergic reactions in some individuals. Pregnant or breastfeeding women should avoid blue vervain due to its potential to stimulate uterine contractions. As with any herbal remedy, it's important to consult with a healthcare provider before using blue vervain, especially if you have underlying health conditions or are taking medications.

Bladderwrack:

Definition: Bladderwrack is a type of seaweed or marine algae commonly used in traditional medicine and as a dietary supplement. It's known for its potential health benefits, particularly related to thyroid health and weight management.

Ingredients: Bladderwrack contains various nutrients, including iodine, vitamins, minerals, and antioxidants. The primary active components are iodine and fucoidan, a type of carbohydrate found in brown seaweeds.

How to Prepare: Bladderwrack supplements are available in various forms, including capsules, powders, and liquid extracts. They can be taken orally with water or added to smoothies and other beverages.

Dosage: The appropriate dosage of bladderwrack can vary based on factors such as age, health status, and the specific product being used. It's essential to follow the recommended dosage on the product label or consult with a healthcare professional for personalized guidance.

How to Use: Bladderwrack supplements are typically taken orally, either with water or mixed into food or beverages. It's important to follow the instructions on the product label and avoid exceeding the recommended dosage.

Side Effects: While bladderwrack is generally considered safe for most people when used in moderation, excessive intake of iodine from bladderwrack supplements can cause thyroid dysfunction and other adverse effects. Individuals with thyroid disorders, iodine sensitivity, or certain medical conditions should exercise caution and consult with a healthcare provider before using bladderwrack supplements. Common side effects may include digestive upset, allergic reactions, or interactions with medications.

Goldenseal:

Definition: Goldenseal, scientifically known as Hydrastis canadensis, is a perennial herb native to North America. It has a long history of use in traditional Native American medicine and later in folk medicine for its potential health benefits.

Ingredients: Goldenseal root contains various bioactive compounds, including alkaloids (such as berberine and hydrastine), flavonoids, and volatile oils. These compounds are believed to contribute to the herb's medicinal properties, including its potential as an antimicrobial, anti-inflammatory, and immune enhancer.

How to Prepare: Goldenseal is typically consumed as an herbal tea, tincture, or in supplement form (such as capsules or tablets). To make tea, dried goldenseal root or leaves are steeped in hot water for several minutes before being strained and consumed.

Dosage: The appropriate dosage of goldenseal can vary depending on factors such as age, health status, and the specific preparation being used. It's important to follow the recommended dosage on the product label or consult with a qualified herbalist or healthcare professional for personalized guidance.

How to Use: Goldenseal tea, tincture, or supplements are typically taken orally. It's often used to support immune function, promote digestive health, and soothe inflammation.

Side Effects: Goldenseal is generally considered safe for most people when used in moderate amounts. However, some individuals may experience mild side effects such as gastrointestinal upset or allergic reactions. It may also interact with certain medications or have adverse effects in individuals with certain health conditions, such as high blood pressure or pregnancy. It's important to use goldenseal under the guidance of a healthcare professional and to discontinue use if any adverse effects occur.

Hops:

Definition: Hops, scientifically known as Humulus lupulus, is a perennial climbing vine native to Europe, Asia, and North America. It is primarily known for its use in brewing beer but has also been used historically in traditional medicine for its potential health benefits.

Ingredients: Hops flowers contain various bioactive compounds, including bitter acids (such as humulone and lupulone), essential oils, flavonoids, and polyphenols. These compounds are believed to contribute to the herb's medicinal properties, including its potential as a sedative, relaxant, and digestive aid.

How to Prepare: Hops is typically consumed as an herbal tea, tincture, or in supplement form (such as capsules or tablets). To make tea, dried hops flowers are steeped in hot water for several minutes before being strained and consumed.

Dosage: The appropriate dosage of hops can vary depending on factors such as age, health status, and the specific preparation being used. It's important to follow the recommended dosage on the product label or consult with a qualified herbalist or healthcare professional for personalized guidance.

How to Use: Hops tea, tincture, or supplements are typically taken orally. It's often used to promote relaxation, relieve anxiety, and support sleep.

Side Effects: Hops is generally considered safe for most people when used in moderate amounts. However, some individuals may experience mild side effects such as drowsiness, gastrointestinal upset, or allergic reactions. It may also interact with certain medications or have adverse effects in individuals with certain health conditions, such as depression or hormone-sensitive conditions. It's important to use hops under the guidance of a healthcare professional and to discontinue use if any adverse effects occur.

Kelp:

Definition: Kelp refers to several species of large brown algae belonging to the Laminariales order. It is commonly found in underwater forests along rocky coastlines around the world. Kelp has been used for centuries in various cultures, particularly in East Asia, for its nutritional and medicinal properties.

Ingredients: Kelp is rich in various nutrients, including iodine, vitamins (such as vitamin K, vitamin C, and B vitamins), minerals (including calcium, magnesium, and potassium), antioxidants, and fiber. These nutrients are believed to contribute to the seaweed's potential health benefits, including its role in thyroid function, bone health, and immune support.

How to Prepare: Kelp is typically consumed dried, powdered, or in supplement form (such as capsules or tablets). It can also be used in cooking, particularly in soups, salads, and stir-fries. Kelp supplements are available in various forms, including powdered extracts, tablets, and liquid extracts.

Dosage: The appropriate dosage of kelp can vary depending on factors such as age, health status, and the specific preparation being used. It's important to follow the recommended dosage on the product label or consult with a qualified healthcare professional for personalized guidance.

How to Use: Kelp supplements are typically taken orally with water. They can be consumed as part of a daily nutritional regimen to support overall health and well-being. Kelp can also be incorporated into recipes as a flavorful and nutritious ingredient.

Side Effects: While kelp is generally considered safe for most people when consumed in moderate amounts, excessive intake of iodine-rich foods or supplements, including kelp, can lead to thyroid dysfunction or iodine toxicity. Some individuals may also be allergic to seaweed and experience allergic reactions. Pregnant or breastfeeding individuals should consult with a healthcare professional before using kelp supplements. It's important to use kelp under the guidance of a healthcare professional and to discontinue use if any adverse effects occur.

THE END